Important Special Notice:

Throughout this book, we made last-minute changes to suggest that persons suspecting contact with anthrax spores should wash first with water only and avoid the use of soap until spores are removed, then wash with soap if desired. We made this suggestion based on studies cited by biological warfare epidemiologist Meryl Nass, M.D., in Appendix 3 and on her website at www.anthraxvaccine.org, which appear to show that soap and detergent substances can increase the virulence of anthrax spores. Although we have also included some government documents which suggest washing with soap and water, we strongly urge review of Dr. Nass' comments in Appendix 3 and on her website before using soap.

Anthrax:

A Practical Guide for Citizens

What You Should Know, What You Can Do, & How It Came to This

a compilation of public materials
intended to serve as a practical citizen's guide

by
The Parents' Committee
for Public Awareness

Harvard Perspectives in Current Affairs
Harvard Perspectives Press

Published and distributed by
Harvard Perspectives Press
Harvard Perspectives in Current Affairs
Belmont, Massachusetts
Email: harvardperspecpr@aol.com

The Parents' Committee for Public Awareness

Anthrax, A Practical Guide for Citizens: What You Should Know, What You Can Do, & How It Came to This

ISBN 0-9715778-0-3

FIRST EDITION, October 2001.

Manufactured in the United States of America.

For M., K., and D.

With hope that yours can be

A safer world

Foreword

In the days after the world changed on September 11, 2001, many of us in America began to cast around for positive things that we could do. Some people enlisted in the military, some marched for peace, some gave blood, some went to New York to help in the work to be done there. Julia Roberts made a public service announcement and Paul McCartney pulled together, with a little help from his friends, a concert. We all had things to do, and it is important that we did them. As parents, a few of us wanted to do something concrete that could help provide information that would be useful to a variety of people including those who care for our children and try to keep them healthy. As the news about anthrax became a bit more grim each day, we decided to pull together this book, also with a little help from our friends, and ultimately we decided to publish it. We hope it will help provide useful information to people in a variety of settings as we all face a terrible terrain that few of us ever expected we would encounter.

We have drawn upon a wide array of public sources, books, and journals for the information presented here, and although most of us are not medical professionals or scientists we have checked and double-checked painstakingly to assure that the information provided here is accurate.   We encourage feedback to our publishers' email address printed on the copyright page, and if there is sufficient interest to update and revise in the future we will certainly try to incorporate such feedback into that effort.

We finally wish to extend our sincere appreciation to biological warfare epidemiologist Meryl Nass, M.D., who has allowed us to draw upon her expertise and writings in this work. Dr. Nass has long been a courageous and straightforward voice both in pointing out and advocating for the necessary steps to make our nation and the world a safer place in the face of the horrors implicit in these pages, and we salute her.

The Parents Committee for Public Awareness

October, 2001

Table of Contents

Appendices

I

WHAT TO DO IF YOU SUSPECT

YOU HAVE BEEN EXPOSED TO ANTHRAX

Do not panic. Use this chapter as a step-by-step guide.

Do not minimize your risk or think "this could never happen to me." The world has changed, and it could happen to almost anyone.

If you suspect that you are in the presence of a package that could contain Anthrax, do not call out to others nearby to come and help you. If you are holding it, gently put it down. Get up and walk away from it, and urge anyone else nearby to do the same. Make sure that it is isolated and the immediate area cordoned off. Do not touch anyone. Ensure that anyone who has touched the package washes their hands and all unprotected skin **with water** for at least 20 seconds per skin surface. **Do not use soap**. If the powder or material is on you or your clothes, change your clothes and shower, placing your clothes in a sealable plastic bag. Notify your local law enforcement authorities. List all persons who have touched the letter and/or envelope. Include contact information and have this information available for the authorities.

Beware of government or media spokespersons who put out simplistic generalizations such as **Newsweek**'s recent claim that "Unless you have recently handled a suspicious package containing a powdery substance, there is no reason to seek out testing." Very few of the dozens of Americans who tested positive for Anthrax exposure in mid-October 2001 had actually handled such packages.

Call your doctor and your family pediatrician.

Doctor's Name:_____

Phone:_____

Pediatrician's Name:_____

Phone:_____

Call other applicable officials, including your workplace supervisor, your local health department, your local police department, and if applicable, your local post office.

Workplace Supervisor:_____

Phone:_____

Local Health Dept:_____

Phone:_____

Local Police Dept:_____

Phone:_____

Local Post Office:_____

Phone:_____

Other Official Contact:_____

Phone:_____

The purpose of these calls is twofold: to get immediate testing and therapeutic intervention for yourself and any family members or associates for whom it is appropriate, and to initiate the appropriate emergency response aimed at helping any other people who may be affected, at preventing others from being exposed, and at tracking down the source of your possible exposure. **When you make these calls, make sure your concerns are treated seriously**.

Get tested, if you suspect you have been exposed to Anthrax. Whether it is a matter of going to your family doctor's office, a local clinic or emergency room, or another site established to respond to a potential crisis, go and get tested at the first opportunity. Tests may include nasal swabs (which are a kind of first take, but not finally conclusive), blood tests (far more accurate), and other procedures. Ask the questions you need to ask to make sure you understand the nature of the tests and what follow-ups may be needed.

Take the antibiotics. If you believe you have been exposed to Anthrax, you need to begin antibiotic treatment immediately and continue it under the care of your physician, either until you have completed the course of treatment (usually 8 weeks to 60 days) or until tests have proven conclusively that you are not infected with Anthrax. Do not take the antibiotics as a preventive measure without getting tested, and do not end the treatment process without a clear and concrete reason for doing so. Indiscriminate use of antibiotics will likely lead to resistant strains of bacteria.

Ciprofloxacin is effective with all known forms of Anthrax, but tetracycline (such as doxycyclin) and penicillin are also effective with most forms of Anthrax and may be cheaper and easier to get. The only form of ciprofloxacin available in the United States at the time of this publication is Cipro, the brand-name version, manufactured by the German company Bayer, which holds the patent and has been fighting possible moves to over-ride the patent so as to allow other companies to begin manufacturing ciprofloxacin. Depending on the progress of this struggle, generic forms of the ciprofloxacin antibiotic may be available in the United States early in 2002. They may already be available in Canada, which moved on October 18, 2001 to over-ride the Bayer patent.

This is an official
CDC Health Advisory

Distributed via Health Alert Network
October 18, 2001

HAND-HELD IMMUNOASSAYS FOR DETECTION OF *Bacillus anthracis* SPORES

Hand-held assays (sometimes referred to as "Smart Tickets") are sold commercially for the rapid detection of *Bacillus anthracis*. These assays are intended only for the screening of environmental samples. First responder and law enforcement communities are using these as instant screening devices and should forward any positive samples to authorities for more sensitive and specialized confirmatory testing. The results of these assays should not be used to make decisions about patient management or prophylaxis. The utility and validity of these assays are unknown.

At this time, CDC does not have enough scientific data to recommend the use of these assays. The analytical sensitivity of these assays is limited by the technology, and data provided by manufacturers indicate that a minimum of 10,000 spores is required to generate a positive signal. This number of spores would suggest a heavy contamination of the area (sample). Therefore a negative result does not rule out a lower level of contamination. Data collected from field use also indicate specificity problems with some of these assays. Some positive results have been obtained with spores of the non-anthrax *Bacillus* bacteria that may be found in the environment.
For these reasons, CDC has been asked to evaluate the sensitivity and specificity of the commercially available rapid, hand-held assays for *B. anthracis*. When this study is completed, results will be made available. Conclusions from this study are not expected in the near future.

II

WHAT TO DO IF YOU RECEIVE AN ENVELOPE OR PACKAGE SUSPECTED TO CONTAIN ANTHRAX OR OTHER BIOLOGICAL AGENTS

DO NOT PANIC.

1. Anthrax organisms can cause skin infection, gastrointestinal infection or pulmonary infection. To do so the organism must be rubbed into abraded skin, swallowed, or inhaled as a fine, aerosolized mist. **It does not leap into one's body**. All forms of disease are generally treatable with antibiotics.

2. For anthrax to be inhaled and enter the lungs, it must be "aerosolized" into particles between 0.4 and 2/10,000ths of an inch, smaller than a red blood cell. It would require a great deal of technical skill and special equipment to render anthrax in such a form. If such small particles are inhaled, life-threatening lung infection can occur, but prompt recognition of exposure and

19

initiation of antibiotics before onset of symptoms should prevent infection.

3. Anthrax is not communicable. It cannot be transferred from one person to another.

If you receive an unopened letter or a letter that appears empty:

1. Place envelope in a plastic bag or glassine envelope

2. Wash hands with WATER for at least 20 seconds. Do not use SOAP.

3. NOTIFY the FBI, State police, and your supervisor (if you are at work).

If you receive an envelope with powder and powder spills out onto surface:

1. DO NOT clean powder up. Keep others away.

2. Wash hands with WATER for at least 20 seconds. Do not use SOAP.

3. DO NOT brush off your clothes.

4. NOTIFY the FBI, state police, and your supervisor.

5. REMOVE clothing and place in plastic bag, as soon as possible.

6. SHOWER with WATER. DO NOT use soap, bleach or other disinfectant

7. PUT on fresh clothing.

8. MAKE list of all people who had contact with the powder and give to local public health authorities. They may be instructed to get tested or to watch for fever or other symptoms over the next couple of days.

If you receive a suspicious package, a package marked with a threatening message, a package without a return address, or a package from a source with which you are unfamiliar:

1. DO NOT OPEN.

2. LEAVE it and EVACUATE the room.

3. KEEP others from entering.

4. NOTIFY the FBI, State police, and your supervisor.

If there is aerosolization or a small explosion:

1. TURN OFF local fans or ventilations units in the area.

2. LEAVE room immediately.

3. CLOSE the door, or section off the area to prevent others from entering.

4. NOTIFY the FBI, State police, and your supervisor.

5. REMAIN on premises until responders arrive.

6. SHUT DOWN air handling system in the building, if possible.

6. MAKE list of all people who were in the building at the time and give to local public health authorities. They may be instructed to get tested or to watch for fever or other symptoms over the next couple of days.

How to identify suspicious packages and letters:

- Restrictive markings such as Confidential, Personal, etc.

- Foreign mail, Air Mail or Special Delivery

- Excessive postage

- Handwritten or poorly typed addresses

- Incorrect titles

- Title, but no name

- Mispellings of common words

- Oily stains, discolorations or odor

- No return address

- Excessive weight

- Lopsided or uneven envelope

- Protruding wires or tinfoil

- Excessive securing material such as string or tape

USPS Message to Customers: The Postal Service places the highest priority on the safety of its employees and customers and the security of the U.S. Mail. We are taking every possible measure to assure the safety of all. We are working tirelessly to keep the mail moving and to keep customers and our employees safe and secure.

America's postal employees have done an outstanding job of keeping the mail moving since Sept 11. We have delivered more than 20 billion pieces of mail since the tragedy. It's important to remember that these are isolated incidents.

While we are taking every possible precaution, we understand the importance of America's mail to its people and its economy and we will continue to deliver it.

We are coordinating our efforts with the FBI and the Department of Health and Human Services. Our Chief Postal Inspector is working with the mailing industry to strengthen the security of business mailrooms. We have established a Mail Security Task Force on hazardous biological and chemical materials that will include our unions, management associations, major mailers, and senior postal managers.

Now more than ever, America is depending on the Postal Service to keep the mail moving safely and securely. Everyone needs to mobilize **common sense** in dealing with this unfamiliar situation.

The information below describes how to identify a suspicious mail piece and the procedures to follow:

What constitutes a suspicious letter or parcel? Some typical characteristics which ought to trigger suspicion include letters or parcels that:

Have any powdery substance on the outside. Are unexpected or from someone unfamiliar to you. Have excessive postage, handwritten or poorly typed address, incorrect titles or titles with no name, or misspellings of common words. Are addressed to someone no longer with your organization or are otherwise outdated. Have no return address, or have one that can't be verified as legitimate. Are of unusual weight, given their size, or are lopsided or oddly shaped. Have an unusual amount of tape. Are marked with restrictive endorsements, such as "Personal" or "Confidential." Have strange odors or stains.

What Should I do if I Receive an Anthrax Threat by Mail?

Do not handle the mail piece or package suspected of contamination. Make sure that damaged or suspicious packages are isolated and the immediate area cordoned off. Ensure that all persons who have touched the mail piece wash their hands with soap and water. Notify your local law enforcement authorities. List all persons who have touched the letter and/or envelope. Include contact information and have this information available for the authorities. Place all items worn when in contact with the suspected mail piece in plastic bags and have them available for law enforcement agents. As soon as practical, shower with soap and water. Notify the Center for Disease Control Emergency Response at 770-488-7100 for answers to any questions.

The mail is safe! People shouldn't stop using the mail because of these isolated incidents. The simple act of paying attention to incoming mail will go a long way in keeping it safe and viable. Everyone, in the mailing community, as well as the American public, should exercise common sense.

Additional information is available on the Postal Service's official web site at www.USPS.com

25

III

What is Anthrax?

The disease known as **Anthrax** is an acute bacterial infection caused by the spore-forming organism *Bacillus anthracis*. It is one of the oldest diseases known to man, and through most of its long history it has been associated with agricultural areas and farm life, and carried by wild and domestic hooved, grass-eating animals such as cows, sheep, antelope and goats in Asia, Africa, South America and parts of Europe. Anthrax most commonly occurs in these animals, but it can also occur in humans when they are exposed to infected animals or animal parts, tissue from infected animals, and bacteria cultured from such tissue. Regions of the world without veterinary public health programs report more anthrax in animals than elsewhere.

During the second half of the twentieth century, Anthrax increasingly became known as a potential "weapon of mass destruction" developed and stockpiled for use both by nations and by terrorist groups.

Direct, person-to-person spread of anthrax is impossible. It is not contagious. Human beings can contract the disease only through exposure to the Anthrax bacterium.

Anthrax spores can live in the soil for many decades, and humans can become infected with anthrax by handling products from infected animals or by inhaling anthrax spores from contaminated animal products. Eating undercooked meat from infected animals also can spread the disease. It is rare to find infected animals in the United States.

Doctors can prescribe effective antibiotics for Anthrax. To be effective, treatment should be initiated early. If left untreated, the disease can be fatal, particularly in the case of exposure through inhalation.

An Anthrax vaccine has been licensed for use in humans, but it is not commercially available in the United States. It is reported to be 93 percent effective. It is manufactured and distributed by BioPort Corp. of Lansing, Michigan, is currently available only through the U.S. Department of Defense, and has reportedly been administered to over two million American service members as well as some civilian government employees. It is a cell-free filtrate vaccine, which means it contains no dead or live bacteria in the preparation. Anthrax vaccines intended for animals should not be used in humans. There has been significant controversy about the human anthrax vaccine now in use and its potential side effects, and some evidence has been presented of a possible link between the vaccine and Gulf War Syndrome. To look further into these issues, we suggest that the reader may wish to turn to the Anthrax Vaccine Home Page maintained by Meryl Nass, M.D., at www.anthraxvaccine.org and to the Official Department of Defense Website for the Anthrax Vaccine Immunization Program, at www.anthrax.osd.mil.

In humans, there are three different types of the Anthrax disease, differentiated by the nature of exposure to the Anthrax bacteria:

- In **cutaneous anthrax**, the disease usually begins after exposure of the human skin to the Anthrax organism. Historically, about 95 percent of anthrax infections occurred when the bacterium entered a cut or abrasion on the skin, such as when handling contaminated wool, hides, leather or hair products of infected animals.   In this type of exposure, itching occurs first, followed by appearance of a skin lesion, usually on the heads, forearms, or hands. The lesion first appears as a small bump resembling an insect bite, then turns into a painless ulcer (one to three centimeters in diameter) and in two to six days develops a black center. It is rarely painful, but can have associated swelling in lymph glands in the affected area. If untreated the infection can spread and cause blood poisoning. Without antibiotics, the mortality rate for cutaneous anthrax has been reported to be as high as 20%; with antibiotics, death due to cutaneous anthrax is rare.

- In **inhalation anthrax**, the disease usually begins after a person has inhaled tiny airborne particles of the bacterium. Initial symptoms of **Inhalation Anthrax** are mild and non-specific, and may resemble a common cold or flu with characteristics of fever, tiredness, mild cough or chest pain. This initial period is followed by a second phase with breathing problems and shock after several days. This second phase is characterized by acute respiratory distress, sepsis and acute haemorrhagic mediastinitis causing mediastinal widening on chest X-ray. In a previously healthy patient, such an X-ray indication of mediastinal widening is highly suggestive of Anthrax. If the disease progresses to this stage it is often fatal.

- **Intestinal Anthrax** is a very rare form of food poisoning that may follow the consumption of contaminated meat. Initial signs include nausea, loss of appetite, vomiting and fever, followed by abdominal pain, vomiting blood and severe diarrhea. It is very difficult to recognize or diagnose and, if untreated, is often fatal.

It is worth noting here that a significant percentage of those exposed to the anthrax bacterium, either by inhalation or cutaneous means, will not become infected. "It takes the inhalation of hundreds of thousand to millions of spores of anthrax to cause the disease inhalation anthrax, with the possible exception of people with immune deficiencies, for whom less spores might lead to illness," according to Dr. Meryl Nass, a practicing physician who is an expert on anthrax, in a memorandum posted October 14, 2001 on her Anthrax Vaccine Home Page web site. "Fewer spores do not cause illness; the immune system seems to readily defend against them. This is presumably why five others in Florida have now been found with anti-anthrax antibodies, but were not ill. In goat hair mills, where workers were daily exposed to anthrax spores, some developed antibodies and some did not."

IV

Antibiotic Treatment and Therapy

Three types of antiobiotics are approved by the U.S. Food and Drug Association for anthrax: ciprofloxacin, tetracyclines (including doxycycline), and penicillins. For people who have been exposed to anthrax but do not have symptoms, 60 days of one of these antibiotics is given to reduce the risk or progression of disease due to inhaled anthrax.

In a document dated October 10, 2001, the U.S. Department of Health and Human Services assured the American public that "under emergency plans, the Federal government would ship appropriate antibiotics from its stockpile to wherever they are needed."

In the meantime, according to the Health and Human Services statement, Cipro should not be prescribed unless there is a clearly indicated need, so that the drug will be available as the need arises for the standard infections for which it is used:

"Although FDA does not regulate the practice of medicine, the agency is strongly recommending that physicians not prescribe Cipro for individual patients to have on hand for possible use against inhaled anthrax. In addition to the potential influence on supply of the drug, indiscriminate prescribing and widespread use of Cipro could hasten the development of drug-resistant organisms."

Cipro has been associated with a number of negative side effects, including significant gastrointestinal distress. Children are particularly susceptible to side effects from Cipro, including joint damage. Cipro should never be taken by pregnant women or women who are breastfeeding.

If you suspect you have been exposed to Anthrax, you need to begin antiobiotic treatment immediately and continue it under the care of your physician, either until you have completed the course of treatment (usually 8 weeks to 60 days) or until tests have proven conclusively that you are not infected with Anthrax. Do not self-medicate as a preventive measure without getting tested, and do not end the treatment process without a clear and concrete reason for doing so.

Ciprofloxacin is effective with all known forms of Anthrax, but tetracycline (such as doxycyclin) and penicillin are also effective with most forms of Anthrax and may be cheaper and easier to get. The only form of ciprofloxacin available in the United States at the time of this publication is Cipro, the brand-name version, manufactured by the German company Bayer, which holds the patent and has been fighting possible moves to over-ride the patent so as to allow other companies to begin manufacturing ciprofloxacin. Depending on the progress of this struggle, generic forms of the ciprofloxacin antibiotic may be available in the United States early in 2002. They may already be available in Canada, which moved on October 18, 2001 to over-ride the Bayer patent.

As of the date of this publication, there were conflicting reports from media, the government, Bayer and other drug companies, and medical professionals as to the adequacy of the supply of any form of ciprofloxacin on hand, in production, or in

planned production.

CDC's National Pharmaceutical Stockpile

A decision to deploy the stockpile is based on the best epidemiologic, laboratory and public health information regarding the nature of the threat.

· The mission of CDC's National Pharmaceutical Stockpile program (NPSP) is to ensure the availability of life saving pharmaceuticals, antibiotics, chemical interventions, as well as medical, surgical and patient support supplies, and equipment for prompt delivery to the site of a disaster, including a possible biological or chemical terrorist event anywhere in the United States.
· The NPSP is available to supplement the initial response to an incident of biological or chemical terrorism. That response will come from local and state emergency, medical and public health personnel.
· A primary purpose of the NPSP is to provide critical drugs and medical material that would otherwise be unavailable to local communities.
· CDC's NPSP is a unique resource available to all United States public health departments.

Contents of Stockpile
· CDC has established relationships with various national security agencies to facilitate continuous updates and analyses of threat agents and ensure that the NPSP reflects current needs.
· Expert panels convened by CDC prioritized the following biological agents: smallpox, anthrax, pneumonic plague, tularemia, botulinum toxin and viral hemorrhagic fevers.
· Because anthrax, plague and tularemia can be effectively treated with antibiotics that are immediately available, purchasing these products for the NPSP formulary was given first priority.
· The NPSP also has a cache of vaccine available to address smallpox threats.
· In addition to medications and supplies for intravenous administration, the NPS include medical equipment that would be essential for treatment, including airway supplies, bandages and dressings, and other emergency medications. These are items that local clinicians may find in short supply in the event of a terrorism incident.

Components of the National Pharmaceutical Stockpile
· The National Pharmaceutical Stockpile (NPSP) has two basic components. The first component consists of eight 12-hour Push Packages for immediate response. These 12-hour Push Packages are fully stocked, positioned in environmentally controlled and secured warehouses, and ready for immediate deployment to reach any affected area within 12 hours of the federal decision to release the assets.

· A 12-hour push package is a preassembled set of supplies, pharmaceuticals, and medical equipment ready for quick delivery to and use in the field. Each "package" consists of 50 tons of material intended to address a mass casualty incident. These packages will permit emergency medical staff to treat a variety of different agents, since the actual threat may not have been identified at the time of the stockpile deployment.

· The second component is comprised of Vendor Managed Inventory (VMI) material. If the incident requires a larger or mulit-phased response, follow-on VMI Packages will be shipped to arrive within 24 to 36 hours.

· The follow-on VMI packages are comprised of pharmaceuticals and supplies that can be "tailored" to provide pharmaceuticals, supplies and/or products specific for the suspected or confirmed agent or combination of agents

V

Vaccines and Prevention

An Anthrax vaccine has been licensed for use in humans, but it is not commercially available in the United States. It has been reported by the government to be 93 percent effective, but the statistical basis of that claim appears to be very narrow and it has been challenged and estimated to be closer to 70 percent by some at least one expert.

The anthrax vaccine is manufactured and distributed by BioPort Corp. of Lansing, Michigan. It is currently available only through the U.S. Department of Defense, and has reportedly been administered to a large number of American service members as well as some civilian government employees. It is a cell-free filtrate vaccine, which means it contains no dead or live bacteria in the preparation.

Anthrax vaccines intended for animals should not be used in humans.

There has been significant controversy about the human anthrax vaccine now in use and its potential side effects, and some evidence has been presented of a possible link between the vaccine and Gulf War Syndrome. To look further into these issues, we suggest that the reader may wish to turn to the Anthrax Vaccine Home Page maintained by Meryl Nass, M.D., at www.anthraxvaccine.org, to the Official Department of Defense Website for the Anthrax Vaccine Immunization Program, at www.anthrax.osd.mil, and to the U.S. Food and Drug Administration's web page on the subject, at http://www.fda.gov/cber/vaccine/anthrax.htm.

The Health Alert Network (HAN)

A bioterrorist attack, like other health threats, would be detected first at the local level. Health departments throughout the nation must be prepared to detect and respond to those threats.

· The Health Alert Network (HAN) is a nationwide program to establish the communications, information, distance-learning, and organizational infrastructure for a new level of defense against health threats, including the possibility of bioterrorism.

· The HAN will link local health departments to one another and to other organizations critical for preparedness and response: community first-responders, hospital and private laboratories, state health departments, CDC, and other federal agencies

· CDC is leading development of the HAN, in partnership with the National Association of County and City Health Officials (NACCHO), the Association of State and Territorial Health Officials (ASTHO), and other health organizations.

Facts about the HAN system

· High-speed, continuous, secure connection to the Internet, access to public health information, and front-line staff skilled in the use of electronic information and communications technology;

· Distance-learning capacity, via satellite- and Web-based technologies, for continuous upgrading of skills in preparedness for bioterrorism and other health threats;

· Early warning systems, such as broadcast fax, to alert local, state and federal authorities and the media about urgent health threats and about the necessary prevention and response actions; and

· Enable local health officials nationwide to instantaneously access and share disease reports, response plans, and CDC diagnostic and treatment guidelines;

· Strengthen local health departments and their links to critical community health organizations, such as hospitals, laboratories, Emergency Medical Systems (EMS), and clinicians, that need to form a coordinated public health response to bioterrorism.

· Enable local, state, and federal health authorities to communicate and coordinate rapidly and securely with each other and with law enforcement agencies.

42

VI

A Brief History of Bioterrorism

Long before the era of modern microbiology brought the prospect of aerosolized germ warfare to the world of the 20th century, ancient armies used filth, cadavers, animal carcasses and contagion as weapons against each other based on the most rudimentary knowledge of the potential destruction that infectious diseases could bring to one another.

Biological terrorism has been around at least since Persian and Roman warriors deposited rotting animal carcasses into the drinking wells of their adversaries in ancient times. Marauding Tatars ended a long siege of the port of Kaffa on the Black Sea by catapulting bodies of bubonic plague victims over the city walls in 1346, and the ensuing victims' flight may have brought the plague to Western Europe.

On this continent, British forces purposely spread smallpox among the native Indian population, and may have caused a smallpox epidemic among Indian tribes in the Ohio River Valley, by sending smallpox-infested blankets as "gifts" to a coalition of Indian tribes who resisted British authority.

Following the beginning of the modern microbiology in the 19th century, biowarfare began in earnest early in the 20th century. Bacteria associated with anthrax and several other diseases were used by Germany during World War I to infect livestock, contaminate animal feed, and poison horses of opposition cavalries. The Japanese army killed an estimated 10,000 Chinese through biowarfare tactics between 1932 and 1945. In 1969 President Richard Nixon ordered the unilateral dismantling of the United States' offensive bioweapons program after the U.S. military staged more than 200 open-air experiments over a twenty-year period above populated areas from Minneapolis to San Francisco to learn how clouds of bacteria would drift and decay in the environment.

In heroic and delightful turnabout during the Second World War, physicians in an occupied area of Poland actually used a kind of defensive biological warfare effectively against the Nazis.

Understanding that the German army avoided areas with epidemic typhus by using something called the Weil-Felix reaction for diagnosis, the physicians used formalin-killed Proteus OX-19 as a vaccine to induce biological false positive tests for typhus in an area of occupied Poland, and residents there were protected from deportation to concentration camps.

Almost immediately after joining the United States, in 1972, in signing the Biological Weapons Convention – a ban on the development, production, stockpiling, or acquisition of biological weapons – the Soviet Union undertook the largest bioweapons buildup in its history. The Soviets employed over 65,000 researchers and technicians at more than 50 labs and testing sites, cooking up 2,000 strains of anthrax alone and producing 20 tons of smallpox virus each year.

Soon after the collapse of the Soviet Union, the American intelligence community has suggested, some of these researchers and technicians may have taken their expertise, and perhaps some of the deadly materials with which they worked, to Iran, Iraq, China, and North Korea. It is possible that there is a connection between the dispersal of some of these "rogue scientists" and the some of the non-state terrorist groups that have been revealed to possess biological weapons during the past decade.

A chilling, if low-tech, example of bioterrorism on American soil occurred in small-town Oregon in 1984 when members of the Rajneeshee religious group sprinkled salmonella poisoning at 10 restaurant salad bars in their local area and caused over 750 restaurant customers to come down with food poisoning, resulting in 45 hospitalizations. The attack was apparently connected to a failed strategy to influence the outcome of a local election.

A Japanese cult, Aum Shinrikyo, dispersed aerosols of anthrax and botulism throughout Tokyo several times during the mid-1990s but these attacks, for unknown reasons, did not produce any reported illness. This group was also responsible for the release of sarin gas in a Tokyo subway station on March

20, 1995, killing 12 and injuring 5,500. That attack is chronicled in the recently published book ***Underground*** by Japanese writer Karuki Murakami.

As this book is published, the world is facing the first sustained campaign of biological weapon terrorism of the 21st century. It remains to be seen whether evidence will prove to us the connection that we already know, instinctively, must exist between this campaign and the commercial jet attacks of September 11. In the same course of time we will find out whether the phenomenon of anthrax-laced letters delivered through the mail is the main feature of this campaign or just a sinister prelude to something even larger.

VII

Anthrax as a Bio-Terror Weapon

Research on anthrax as a biological weapon began more than 80 years ago during World War I, when Germany sponsored covert efforts among neutral trading partners of the Allies to infect livestock intended for Allied forces. Iraq, in particular, has acknowledged production and weaponizing of anthrax, among other bio- and chemical warfare agents. It is widely believed that Iraq acquired this technology from "rogue" former Soviet Union scientists following the breakup of the Soviet Union.

Despite a widely held belief that any group would need advanced biotechnology to produce a lethal anthrax aerosol, American experts suspect that autonomous groups with substantial funding and contacts could acquire the required materials for a successful attack. An anthrax aerosol would be odorless and invisible following release and would have the potential to travel many miles before disseminating, according to an expert committee brought together by the World Health

Organization in 1970. These experts theorized that the theoretical aircraft release of 50 kg of anthrax over an urban area of 5 million people would results in 250,000 deaths. More recent;y, the U.S. Congressional Office of Technology Assessment estimated that between 130,000 and 3 million deaths could be caused by the aerosolized release of 100 kg of anthrax spores upwind of the Washington, DC area.

Experts have not known what exactly to make of the apparent narrow targeting of news media outlets and political leaders with anthrax-laced "letters" sent through the U.S. mail in September and October 2001. The fact that several individuals have contracted inhalation anthrax suggests, as Dr. Meryl Nass has pointed out, that "there must have been millions more [spores] in the office[s]."

In a later memo on October 21, 2001, Dr. Nass has asked: "Are the anthrax-containing envelopes an initial tease, or warning? They are a good way to disseminate small quantities, while avoiding identification of the sender. But what may be ahead? Spores in ventilation systems? Spores at sports events or where there are dense population concentrations? Thousands or millions of letters containing anthrax? How will we know in time, and how will we decontaminate ventilation systems, electronics, sports arenas, soil, etc.?"

Regarding the shockingly large number of hoaxes reported by law enforcement authorities, Dr. Nass has pointed out that "Hoaxes may also be a strategy of a terrorist. Remember how the anti-ballistic missile program has been criticized for its inability to deal with thousands of dummy missiles which could provide cover for a small number of 'real' missiles? We may be seeing the same thing now."

VIII

Other Bio-Terror Weapons

The following material has been provided by the Centers for Disease Control and updated in September 2001. It outlines the salient facts about the other potential bio-terror weapons currently considered to pose the greatest danger to human beings: botulism, pneumonic plague, and smallpox. We have added information about tularemia from other public sources:

Facts about Botulism

Botulism is a muscle-paralyzing disease caused by a toxin made by a bacterium called *Clostridium botulinum*.

There are three main kinds of botulism:

- Foodborne botulism occurs when a person ingests pre-formed toxin that leads to illness within a few hours to days. Foodborne botulism is a public health emergency because the contaminated food may still be available to

53

other persons besides the patient.

· Infant botulism occurs in a small number of susceptible infants each year who harbor *C. botulinum* in their intestinal tract.

· Wound botulism occurs when wounds are infected with *C. botulinum* that secretes the toxin.

With foodborne botulism, symptoms begin within 6 hours to 2 weeks (most commonly between 12 and 36 hours) after eating toxin-containing food. Symptoms of botulism include double vision, blurred vision, drooping eyelids, slurred speech, difficulty swallowing, dry mouth, muscle weakness that always descends through the body: first shoulders are affected, then upper arms, lower arms, thighs, calves, etc. Paralysis of breathing muscles can cause a person to stop breathing and die, unless assistance with breathing (mechanical ventilation) is provided.

Botulism is not spread from one person to another. Foodborne botulism can occur in all age groups.

A supply of antitoxin against botulism is maintained by CDC. The antitoxin is effective in reducing the severity of symptoms if administered early in the course of the disease. Most patients eventually recover after weeks to months of supportive care.

Facts about Pneumonic Plague

Plague is an infectious disease of animals and humans caused by the bacterium Y*ersinia pestis. Y. pestis*, is found in rodents and their fleas in many areas around the world.

Pneumonic plague occurs when *Y. pestis* infects the lungs. The first signs of illness in pneumonic plague are fever, headache, weakness, and cough productive of bloody or watery sputum. The pneumonia progresses over 2 to 4 days and may cause septic shock and, without early treatment, death.

Person-to-person transmission of pneumonic plague occurs through respiratory droplets, which can only infect those who have face-to-face contact with the ill patient.

Early treatment of pneumonic plague is essential. Several antibiotics are effective, including streptomycin, tetracycline, and chloramphenicol.

There is no vaccine against plague. Prophylactic antibiotic treatment for 7 days will protect persons who have had face-to-face contact with infected patients.

Facts about Smallpox

Smallpox infection killed more than 500 million people during the 20th century before it was eradicated in the late 1970s. The smallpox virus still exists in laboratories in Atlanta and in Koltsovo, Russia, that are overseen by the World Health Organization (WHO), but bioterrorism specialists believe that "rogue scientists" may have sold or made off with secret stores of smallpox when the Soviet Union broke up. A smalpox attack could be particularly devastating because each sneeze or cough could infect dozens of others before recognizable symptoms appear in a carrier.

Smallpox is caused by variola virus. The incubation period is about 12 days (range: 7 to 17 days) following exposure. Initial symptoms include high fever, fatigue, and head and back aches. A characteristic rash, most prominent on the face, arms, and legs, follows in 2-3 days. The rash starts with flat red lesions that evolve at the same rate. Lesions become pus-filled and begin to crust early in the second week. Scabs develop and then separate and fall off after about 3-4 weeks. The majority of patients with smallpox recover, but death occurs in up to 30% of cases.

Smallpox is spread from one person to another by infected saliva droplets that expose a susceptible person having face-to-face contact with the ill person. Persons with smallpox are most infectious during the first week of illness, because that is when the largest amount of virus is present in saliva. However, some risk of transmission lasts until all scabs have fallen off.

Routine vaccination against smallpox ended in 1972. The level of immunity, if any, among persons who were vaccinated before 1972 is uncertain; therefore, these persons are assumed to be susceptible.

Vaccination against smallpox is not recommended to prevent the disease in the general public and therefore is not available.

In people exposed to smallpox, the vaccine can lessen the severity of or even prevent illness if given within 4 days after exposure. Vaccine against smallpox contains another live virus called vaccinia. The vaccine does not contain smallpox virus.

The United States currently has an emergency supply of smallpox vaccine.

There is no proven treatment for smallpox but research to evaluate new antiviral agents is ongoing. Patients with smallpox can benefit from supportive therapy (intravenous fluids, medicine to control fever or pain, etc.) and antibiotics for any secondary bacterial infections that occur.

Facts About Tularemia

Naturally occurring tularemia is a zoonotic disease that is transmitted to humans via contact with infected animals or from the bite of arthropods that have fed on infected animals. It is caused by the highly infectious, slow-growing, aerobic, non-sporulating, Gram negative coccobacillus *Francisella tularensis*. As few as 10-50 organisms are sufficient to cause disease if inhaled or innoculated into the skin. Discovered in the early 20th century, the disease has caused multiple sporadic outbreaks but no large epidemics. During the 1990s, annual incidence has been less than 200 cases nationwide.

Pneumonic tularemia is considered one of the diseases most likely to be encountered in a bioterrorism event. Intentional aerosol release should be suspected if cases occur in nonendemic areas when no discernible risk factors for exposure are identified. Outbreaks of any form of tularemia should be rapidly investigated to rule out a bioterrorism event.

There are six forms of tularemia, classified by clinical presentation and determined by route of exposure:

- **Pneumonic tularemia**. Although up to half of all tularemia cases present with lung involvement from hematogenous spread of systemic infection (secondary pneumonic), this term is generally used to describe infection in the lung as a result of direct inhalation of aerosolized bacteria (primary pneumonic) which is not associated with skin ulcers or lymphadenopathy. Primary pneumonic has accounted for less than 5% of all tularemia cases, but is associated with one of the highest mortality rates when untreated: 30 to 60% of untreated cases have resulted in death. This form is the most likely to be seen in a bioterrorism setting, but can also be seen after the handling of infected animals or contaminated soil.

- **Typhoidal tularemia** presents as severe systemic disease without skin ulcers, lymphadenopathy or pneumonia. Any route of infection possible. Historically has accounted for 5 to 15% of all tularemia cases, with a mortality rate similar to pneumonic. Could be seen in bioterrorism setting, but less likely than pneumonic.

- **Ulceroglandular tularemia.** Characterized by skin ulcer and regional lymphadenopathy. Occurs via contact with an infected animal (particularly rabbits) or by arthropod (particularly tick) bite. Most common natural form of disease, historically accounting for 50 to 85% of cases. Mortality rate for this form has been less than 5%.

- **Glandular tularemia.** Regional lymphadenopathy without a skin ulcer. Approximately 10% of cases. Mortality similar to ulceroglandular.

- **Oculoglandular tularemia.** Conjuctivitis and local lymphadenopathy following innoculation into the eye. Theorteically possible from aerosol or from direct contact with infected material. Has accounted for less than 5% of all cases, with mortality similar to ulceroglandular.

- **Oropharyngeal tularemia.** Pharyngitis and cervical lymphadenopathy following ingestion of inadequately cooked meat from an infected animal. Has accounted for less than 5% of all cases, with mortality similar to ulceroglandular.

Diagnosis. There are currently no widely available rapid confirmatory diagnostic tests for tularemia. A presumptive diagnosis can be made quickly based on presenting symptoms if there is a high index of suspicion. Blood, sputum, biopsy, specimens, pleural fluid, conjunctival exudates and pharyngeal washings may all be obtained to aid in diagnosis.

- **Presumptive diagnosis** can be based on appropriate clinical presentation, especially important in an outbreak setting. Suspicion should be particularly high in the setting of a large number of previously healthy persons presenting with a severe pneumonia with or without skin ulcers and lymphadenopathy, associated with temperature/pulse dissocation and pleural involvement, not responding to typical pneumonia antibiotics. Several tests including fluorescent antibody detection assays, PCR, immunohistochemical stains, and antigen detection assays may be available at reference laboratories.

- **Confirmatory diagnosis**.

  - **Microbiologic**. *F. tularensis* can be cultured from any infected fluids, however the sensitivity is low, even on specific cysteine-enriched media. Also, because of the high risk of exposure to the organism in culture, some microbiology laboratories do not set up cultures if tularemia is suspected. Gram stain is usually negative.

- **Serologic**. Sreum agglutinin antibody assays and enzyme linked immunosorbent assays (ELISA) are of limited use in acute infection because antibody levels are generally not detected until two weeks after infection.

Treatment should be initiated as soon as a diagnosis of tularemia is suspected, and should not be delayed for confirmatory testing. Cure rates are high if antibiotics are started prior to development of severe illness, and survivors have no long-term sequelae. Naturally occurring *F. tularensis* exhibits reliable susceptibility patterns, but unusual resistance patterns could be a concern in a bioterrorism event.

Indicated therapies can include streptomycin or gentamicin. Streptomycin should be avoided in pregnant or lactating women. Alternative therapies include ciprofloxacin, doxycycline, and chloramphenicol.

Post-Exposure Propylaxis. Prophylactic therapy for tularemia should be provided for 14 days for persons who were likely exposed to known intentional release within the last few days, and for laboratory workers with a high risk of expose (e.g., spill of culture, centrifuge aerosolization).

Vaccination. A safe, live attenuated vaccine offering moderate protection versus pneumonic tularemia has been used in the U.S. since 1959 with a very limited availability for laboratory workers at high risk. As tularemia has a short incubation period, and the vaccine has a delayed effect, it is not recommended for post exposure prophylaxis.

Protocols

Interim Recommended Notification Procedures for Local and State Public Health Department Leaders In the Event of a Bioterrorist Incident

	Background	
Local Health Officer is informed of a bioterrorist incident or threat	<<--- OR --->>	Local health officer suspects that cases of illness may be due to a bioterrorist incident

First:
* Notify FBI
* Notify local law enforcement

\ /

First:
Inform & involve State Health Department. Health Department notifies CDC. Conduct investigation.

\ /

Next:
Notify & involve State Health Department and other response partners, per a pre-established notification list

Is BT incident confirmed or thought to be probable?

Yes <--- probable? ---> No

\ /

State Health Department notifies the CDC

Notify FBI. Notify other pre-determined response partners.

Continue investigation.

U.S. Centers for Disease Control

IX

HELPING CHILDREN DEAL WITH CATASTROPHES

In a press release posted on the Brazelton Foundation web site (www.brazelton.org) shortly after the September 11 attacks, noted pediatrician T. Berry Brazelton, MD wrote:

"We are all stunned at the terrible tragedies that happened in New York, Washington, D.C., and Pittsburgh, Pennsylvania. None of us, as parents, can understand why these things happened. We do know that the United States will never be the same again, and we are all frightened and anxious about our country's future.

"As parents, our hearts and minds immediately go to our children. What will this mean to their future? We have been raising our children and grandchildren in a world that has become less and less predictable and increasingly violent. But none of us ever dreamed of such destruction. Many of our children have seen Hollywood versions of such disasters. Now they must wonder about how much they can trust our assurances that 'it's only a movie' and 'it will never happen here.'

"Our children have seen the World Trade Center blown up by terrorists and they have seen the shock and horror on our faces. Now they will need to face the reality of these tragic events and learn to cope with their own fears and concerns. I remember when the space shuttle, Challenger, exploded with Christa McAuliffe aboard. She was a teacher and a mother. Many children wondered, 'Did this happen because she was a bad mother or because her children were bad?'

"In '**Touchpoints: Three to Six**,' the new book I have written with Dr. Joshua Sparrow, a child psychiatrist, we point out that children in this age group tend to take responsibility for such events. They worry that if they are bad, something terrible will happen to their parents too.

"Older children will begin to question a world in which such a horrible event can take place. The impulse control that adolescents and preadolescents are working so hard to master is shaken by their inability to rely on adult models around them. They wonder, 'Will I ever feel safe again?'

"After such a catastrophe, parents need to sit down with their children to share their fears and anxiety. Be ready to listen to what your kids have to say, and be prepared to wait. They may not be ready to share their feelings today or even tomorrow; you may have to wait until next week. Just be sure they know that you are there for them and are ready to answer their questions and discuss their fears whenever they need you. Don't let the defenses of young children fool you. They may say, 'Why are you so upset? It didn't happen to us.' This is just a way to cover up their very real fears and anxiety.

"When your children are ready to talk, you'll likely be asked questions such as, 'Will it happen to me? Will it happen to you? Why did it happen to all those other families?' Be prepared

with answers that are age appropriate. And be ready to share an

older child's anxiety about the kind of world in which we live.

I do not feel we can protect children from these fears and from

our horror, but we can surely share it with them. This is a time

to turn inward, to gather our families, and to talk about our

value systems and our religious beliefs. We must assure children

that we intend to protect ourselves so we can be here for them.

They need to hear that and to believe with us that we can still

believe in the future."

X

Other Resources

Books and Website Addresses

Here are a few books that may be helpful to people

interested in this and related subjects:

Anthrax: The Investigation of a Deadly Outbreak
by Jeanne Guillemin - Paperback - 339 pages (February 5, 2001)
University of California Press; ISBN: 0520229177 List Price:
$17.95

**Chemical and Biological Weapons: Anthrax and Sarin
(High-Tech Military Weapons)** by Gregory Payan Paperback -
259 pages (September 2000) Owl Books; ISBN: 080505765X
List Price: $15.00

**21st Century Bioterrorism and Germ Weapons - U.S. Army
Field Manual for the Treatment of Biological Warfare
Agent Casualties (Anthrax, Smallpox, Plague, Viral Fevers,
Toxins, Delivery Methods, Detection, Symptoms,
Treatment, Equipment)** by Department of Defense Ring-bound -
110 pages (September 30, 2001) Progressive Management;
ISBN: 1931828105 List Price: $29.95

Super Terrorism : Biological, Chemical, and Nuclear by
Yonah Alexander (Editor), Milton M. Hoenig (Editor) Paperback
(August 2001)
Transnational Pub; ISBN: 1571052186 List Price: $35.00

The Biology of Doom : The History of America's Secret Germ Warfare Project by Ed Regis Paperback - 259 pages (September 2000) Owl Books; ISBN: 080505765X List Price: $15.00

Plague Wars : A True Story of Biological Warfare by Tom Mangold, Jeff Goldberg, Goldberg Mangold Hardcover - 336 pages (February 2000)
St. Martin's Press; ISBN: 0312203535 List Price: $27.95

Scourge : The Once and Future Threat of Smallpox by Jonathan B. Tucker
Hardcover - 304 pages (September 2, 2001) Atlantic Monthly Pr; ISBN: 0871138301 List Price: $26.00

First Responder Chem-Bio Handbook by Ben N. Venzke (Editor) Spiral-bound - 198 pages (February 1, 1998) Tempest Publishing; ISBN: 096654370X List Price: $18.00

Combating Chemical, Biological, Radiological, and Nuclear Terrorism : A Comprehensive Strategy : A Report of the Csis Homeland Defense Project) by Frank J. Cilluffo, Sharon L. Cardash, Gordon Nathaniel Lederman Paperback - 72 pages (May 21, 2001) Center for Strategic & Int'l Studies; ISBN: 0892063890 List Price: $19.95

Jane's Chem-Bio Handbook by Frederick R. Sidell Paperback Spiral edition (February 1998) Jane's Information Group; ISBN: 0710619235
List Price: $32.50

Chem-Bio: Frequently Asked Questions by Barbara Graves (Editor)
Paperback - 175 pages 1 edition (September 1998) Tempest Publishing; ISBN: 0966543718 List Price: $18.00

Germs: Biological Weapons and America's Secret War by Judith Miller, Stephen Engelberg, William J. Broad Hardcover - 352 pages (September 2001) Simon & Schuster; ISBN: 0684871580 List Price: $27.00

The Coming Plague : Newly Emerging Diseases in a World Out of Balance by Laurie Garrett Paperback Reprint edition (October 1995) Penguin USA (Paper); ISBN: 0140250913 List Price: $15.95

Usama bin Laden's al-Qaida: Profile of a Terrorist Network by Yonah Alexander, Michael S. Swetnam **Paperback** (April 2001) Transnational Pub; ISBN: 1571052194 **List Price:** $17.50

Toxic Terror (BCSIA Studies in International Security) by Jonathan B. Tucker (Editor) Paperback - 320 pages (February 25, 2000)   MIT Press; ISBN: 0262700719 **List Price:** $20.00

Underground (Vintage International) by Haruki Murakami Paperback - 366 pages (April 10, 2001) Vintage Books; ISBN: 0375725806 List Price: $14.00

In addition, to keep up to date with rapidly changing developments and news on Anthrax and the other topics with which it is inextricably related, we suggest the following sites on the world wide web:

Centers for Disease Control: http://www.bt.cdc.gov/

U.S. Dept. of Defense; Nuclear, Biological, Chemical Medical Reference Site: http://www.nbc-med.org/others/

Journal of the American Medical Association (Scroll down a screen or two to see this message: **Articles on Bioterrorism**

Five articles on bioterrorism by the Working Group on Civilian Biodefense—addressing anthrax, smallpox, plague, botulinum toxin, and tularemia—are online and free of charge. In addition, the *JAMA* theme issue on Bioterrorism is online and free of charge. On October 19, the CDC published reports related to the recent cases of anthrax in the United States in *MMWR*. These articles also will be published in the November 7 issue of *JAMA*.) http://jama.ama-assn.org/

World Health Organization web site on "Responding to the deliberate use of biological agents and chemicals as weapons" at http://www.who.int/emc/deliberate_epi.html.

Epidemiologist Meryl Nass, M.D., maintains an extremely helpful website called the Anthrax Vaccine Home Page at www.anthraxvaccine.org. **She can also be reached my mail at Meryl Nass, M.D., 124 Wardtown Road, Freeport, Maine 04032 and by telephone at 207-865-7000.**

The Center for the Study of Bioterrorism and Emerging Infections of the Saint Louis University, School of Public Health: http://www.slu.edu/colleges/sph/bioterrorism/index.html

This last site is remarkably inclusive, well-organized, and up-to-date. Rather than provide a long list of web addresses that will likely go through myriad changes and required regular updating, we strongly suggest that interested readers focus on the The Center for the Study of Bioterrorism and Emerging Infections of the Saint Louis

University, School of Public Health and use it to organize

online research. This site's "Internet Resources" tab is

subdivided into the categories of Government Resources,

Professional Organization Resources, Academic

Resources, State Health Departments, Centers for Public

Health Preparedness, and Veterinary Resources.

Appendix 1:

Recognition of Illness Associated with the Intentional Release

of a Biologic Agent

US Centers for Disease Control, Morbidity and Mortality Weekly Report, October 18, 2001
http://www.cdc.gov/mmwr/preview/mmwrhtml/mm5041a2.htm

On September 11, 2001, following the terrorist incidents in New York City and Washington, D.C., CDC recommended heightened surveillance for any unusual disease occurrence or increased numbers of illnesses that might be associated with the terrorist attacks. Subsequently, cases of anthrax in Florida and New York City have demonstrated the risks associated with intentional release of biologic agents (*1*). This report provides guidance for health-care providers and public health personnel about recognizing illnesses or patterns of illness that might be associated with intentional release of biologic agents.

Health-Care Providers

Health-care providers should be alert to illness patterns and diagnostic clues that might indicate an unusual infectious disease outbreak associated with intentional release of a biologic agent and should report any clusters or findings to their local or state health department. The covert release of a biologic agent may not have an immediate impact because of the delay between exposure and illness onset, and outbreaks associated with intentional releases might closely resemble naturally occurring outbreaks. Indications of intentional release of a biologic agent include 1) an unusual temporal or geographic clustering of illness (e.g., persons who attended the same public event or gathering) or patients presenting with clinical signs and symptoms that suggest an infectious disease outbreak (e.g., ≥ 2 patients presenting with an unexplained febrile illness associated with sepsis, pneumonia, respiratory failure, or rash or a botulism-like syndrome with flaccid muscle paralysis, especially if occurring in otherwise healthy persons); 2) an unusual age distribution for common diseases (e.g., an increase in what appears to be a chickenpox-like illness among adult patients, but which might be smallpox); and 3) a large number of cases of acute flaccid paralysis with prominent bulbar palsies, suggestive of a release of *botulinum* toxin.

CDC defines three categories of biologic agents with potential to be used as weapons, based on ease of dissemination or transmission, potential for major public health impact (e.g., high mortality), potential for public panic and social disruption, and requirements for public health preparedness (*2*). Agents of highest concern are *Bacillus anthracis* (anthrax), *Yersinia pestis* (plague), variola major (smallpox), *Clostridium botulinum* toxin (botulism), *Francisella tularensis* (tularemia), filoviruses (Ebola hemorrhagic fever, Marburg hemorrhagic fever); and arenaviruses (Lassa [Lassa fever], Junin [Argentine hemorrhagic fever], and related viruses). The following summarizes the clinical features of these agents (*3--6*).

Anthrax. A nonspecific prodrome (i.e., fever, dyspnea, cough, and chest discomfort) follows inhalation of infectious spores. Approximately 2--4 days after initial symptoms, sometimes after a brief period of improvement, respiratory failure and hemodynamic collapse ensue. Inhalational anthrax also might include thoracic edema and a widened mediastinum on chest radiograph. Gram-positive bacilli can grow on blood culture, usually 2--3 days after onset of illness. Cutaneous anthrax follows deposition of the organism onto the skin, occurring particularly on exposed areas of the hands, arms, or face. An area of local edema becomes a pruritic macule or papule, which enlarges and ulcerates after 1--2 days. Small, 1--3 mm vesicles may surround the ulcer. A painless, depressed, black eschar usually with surrounding local edema subsequently develops. The syndrome also may include lymphangitis and painful lymphadenopathy.

Plague. Clinical features of pneumonic plague include fever, cough with muco-purulent sputum (gram-negative rods may be seen on gram stain), hemoptysis, and chest pain. A chest radiograph will show evidence of bronchopneumonia.

Botulism. Clinical features include symmetric cranial neuropathies (i.e., drooping eyelids, weakened jaw clench, and difficulty swallowing or speaking), blurred vision or diplopia, symmetric descending weakness in a proximal to distal pattern, and respiratory dysfunction from respiratory muscle paralysis or upper airway obstruction without sensory deficits. Inhalational botulism would have a similar clinical presentation as foodborne botulism; however, the gastrointestinal symptoms that accompany foodborne botulism may be absent.

Smallpox (variola). The acute clinical symptoms of smallpox resemble other acute viral illnesses, such as influenza, beginning with a 2--4 day nonspecific prodrome of fever and myalgias before rash onset. Several clinical features can help clinicians differentiate varicella (chickenpox) from smallpox. The rash of varicella is most prominent on the trunk and develops in successive groups of lesions over several days, resulting in lesions in various stages of development and resolution. In comparison, the vesicular/pustular rash of smallpox is typically most prominent on the face and extremities, and lesions develop at the same time.

Inhalational tularemia. Inhalation of *F. tularensis* causes an abrupt onset of an acute, nonspecific febrile illness beginning 3--5 days after exposure, with pleuropneumonitis developing in a substantial proportion of cases during subsequent days (*7*).

Hemorrhagic fever (such as would be caused by Ebola or Marburg viruses). After an incubation period of usually 5--10 days (range: 2--19 days), illness is characterized by abrupt onset of fever, myalgia, and headache. Other signs and symptoms include nausea and vomiting, abdominal pain, diarrhea, chest pain, cough, and pharyngitis. A maculopapular rash, prominent on the trunk, develops in most patients approximately 5 days after onset of illness. Bleeding manifestations, such as petechiae, ecchymoses, and hemorrhages, occur as the disease progresses (*8*).

Clinical Laboratory Personnel

Although unidentified gram-positive bacilli growing on agar may be considered as contaminants and discarded, CDC recommends that these bacilli be treated as a "finding" when they occur in a suspicious clinical setting (e.g., febrile illness in a previously healthy person). The laboratory should attempt to characterize the organism, such as motility testing, inhibition by penicillin, absence of hemolysis on sheep blood agar, and further biochemical testing or species determination.

An unusually high number of samples, particularly from the same biologic medium (e.g., blood and stool cultures), may alert laboratory personnel to an outbreak. In addition, central laboratories that receive clinical specimens from several sources should be alert to increases in demand or unusual requests for culturing (e.g., uncommon biologic specimens such as cerebrospinal fluid or pulmonary aspirates).

When collecting or handling clinical specimens, laboratory personnel should 1) use Biological Safety Level II (BSL-2) or Level III (BSL-3) facilities and practices when working with clinical samples considered potentially infectious; 2) handle all specimens In a BSL-2 laminar flow hood with protective eyewear (e.g., safety glasses or eye shields), use closed-front laboratory coats with cuffed sleeves, and stretch the gloves over the cuffed sleeves; 3) avoid any activity that places persons at risk for infectious exposure, especially activities that might create aerosols or droplet dispersal; 4) decontaminate laboratory benches after each use and dispose of supplies and equipment in proper receptacles; 5) avoid touching mucosal surfaces with their hands (gloved or ungloved), and never eat or drink in the laboratory; and 6) remove and reverse their gloves before leaving the laboratory and dispose of them in a biohazard container, and wash their hands and remove their laboratory coat.

When a laboratory is unable to identify an organism in a clinical specimen, it should be sent to a laboratory where the agent can be characterized, such as the state public health laboratory or, in some large metropolitan areas, the local health department laboratory. Any clinical specimens suspected to contain variola (smallpox) should be reported to local and state health authorities and then transported to CDC. All variola diagnostics should be conducted at CDC laboratories. Clinical laboratories should report any clusters or findings that could indicate intentional release of a biologic agent to their state and local health departments.

Infection-Control Professionals

Heightened awareness by infection-control professionals (ICPs) facilitates recognition of the release of a biologic agent. ICPs are involved with many aspects of hospital operations and several departments and with counterparts in other hospitals. As a result, ICPs may recognize changing patterns or clusters in a hospital or in a community that might otherwise go unrecognized.

ICPs should ensure that hospitals have current telephone numbers for notification of both internal (ICPs, epidemiologists, infectious diseases specialists, administrators, and public affairs officials) and external (state and local health departments, Federal Bureau of Investigation field office, and CDC Emergency Response office) contacts and that they are distributed to the appropriate personnel (*9*). ICPs should work with clinical microbiology laboratories, on- or off-site, that receive specimens for testing from their facility to ensure that cultures from suspicious cases are evaluated appropriately.

State Health Departments

State health departments should implement plans for educating and reminding health-care providers about how to recognize unusual illnesses that might indicate intentional release of a biologic agent. Strategies for responding to potential bioterrorism include 1) providing information or reminders to health-care providers and clinical laboratories about how to report events to the appropriate public health authorities; 2) implementing a 24-hour-a-day, 7-day-a-week capacity to receive and act on any positive report of events that suggest intentional release of a biologic agent; 3) investigating immediately any report of a cluster of illnesses or other event that suggests an intentional release of a biologic agent and requesting CDC's assistance when necessary; 4) implementing a plan, including accessing the Laboratory Response Network for Bioterrorism, to collect and transport specimens and to store them appropriately before laboratory analysis; and 5) reporting immediately to CDC if the results of an investigation suggest release of a biologic agent.

Reported by: National Center for Infectious Diseases; Epidemiology Program Office; Public Health Practice Program Office; Office of the Director, CDC.

Editorial Note:

Health-care providers, clinical laboratory personnel, infection control professionals, and health departments play critical and complementary roles in recognizing and responding to illnesses caused by intentional release of biologic agents. The syndrome descriptions, epidemiologic clues, and laboratory recommendations in this report provide basic guidance that can be implemented immediately to improve recognition of these events.

After the terrorist attacks of September 11, state and local health departments initiated various activities to improve surveillance and response, ranging from enhancing communications (between state and local health departments and between public health agencies and health-care providers) to conducting special surveillance projects. These special projects have included active surveillance for changes in the number of hospital admissions, emergency department visits, and occurrence of specific syndromes. Activities in bioterrorism preparedness and emerging infections over the past few years have better positioned public health agencies to detect and respond to the intentional release of a biologic agent. Immediate review of these activities to identify the most useful and practical approaches will help refine syndrome surveillance efforts in various clinical situations.

Information about clinical diagnosis and management can be found elsewhere (*1--9*). Additional information about responding to bioterrorism is available from CDC at <http://www.bt.cdc.gov>; the U.S. Army Medical Research Institute of Infectious Diseases at <http://www.usamriid.army.mil/education/bluebook.html>; the Association for Infection Control Practitioners at <http://www.apic.org>; and the Johns Hopkins Center for Civilian Biodefense at <http://www.hopkins-biodefense.org>.

References

1. CDC. Update: investigation of anthrax associated with intentional exposure and interim public health guidelines, October 2001. MMWR 2001;50:889--93.
2. CDC. Biological and chemical terrorism: strategic plan for preparedness and response. MMWR 2000;49(no. RR-4).
3. Arnon SS, Schechter R, Inglesby TV, et al. Botulinum toxin as a biological weapon: medical and public health management. JAMA 2001;285:1059--70.
4. Inglesby TV, Dennis DT, Henderson DA, et al. Plague as a biological weapon: medical and public health management. JAMA 2000;283:2281--90.
5. Henderson DA, Inglesby TV, Bartlett JG, et al. Smallpox as a biological weapon: medical and public health management. JAMA 1999;281:2127--37.
6. Inglesby TV, Henderson DA, Bartlett JG, et al. Anthrax as a biological weapon: medical and public health management. JAMA 1999;281:1735--963.

7. Dennis DT, Inglesby TV, Henderson DA, et al. Tularemia as a biological weapon: medical and public health management. JAMA 2001;285:2763--73.
8. Peters CJ. Marburg and Ebola virus hemorrhagic fevers. In: Mandell GL, Bennett JE, Dolin R, eds. Principles and practice of infectious diseases. 5th ed. New York, New York: Churchill Livingstone 2000;2:1821--3.
9. APIC Bioterrorism Task Force and CDC Hospital Infections Program Bioterrorism Working Group. Bioterrorism readiness plan: a template for healthcare facilities. Available at <http://www.cdc.gov/ncidod/hip/Bio/bio.htm>. Accessed October 2001.

Appendix 2

Update: Investigation of Anthrax Associated with Intentional Exposure and Interim Public Health Guidelines, October 2001

US Centers for Disease Control, Morbidity and Mortality Weekly Report, October 19, 2001   50(41);889-893
http://www.cdc.gov/mmwr/preview/mmwrhtml/mm5041a1.htm

On October 4, 2001, CDC and state and local public health authorities reported a case of inhalational anthrax in Florida (*1*). Additional cases of anthrax subsequently have been reported from Florida and New York City. This report updates the findings of these case investigations, which indicate that infections were caused by the intentional release of *Bacillus anthracis*. This report also includes interim guidelines for postexposure prophylaxis for prevention of inhalational anthrax and other information to assist epidemiologists, clinicians, and laboratorians responding to intentional anthrax exposures.

For these investigations, a confirmed case of anthrax was defined as 1) a clinically compatible case of cutaneous, inhalational, or gastrointestinal illness* that is laboratory confirmed by isolation of *B. anthracis* from an affected tissue or site or 2) other laboratory evidence of *B. anthracis* infection based on at least two supportive laboratory tests. A suspected case was defined as 1) a clinically compatible case of illness without isolation of *B. anthracis* and no alternative diagnosis, but with laboratory evidence of *B. anthracis* by one supportive laboratory test or 2) a clinically compatible case of anthrax epidemiologically linked to a confirmed environmental exposure, but without corroborative laboratory evidence of *B. anthracis* infection.

Laboratory criteria for diagnosis of anthrax consist of 1) isolation and confirmation of *B. anthracis* from a clinical specimen collected from an affected tissue or site or 2) other supportive laboratory tests, including (a) evidence of *B. anthracis* DNA by polymerase chain reaction (PCR) from specimens collected from an affected tissue or site, (b) demonstration of *B. anthracis* in a clinical specimen by immunohistochemical staining, or (c) other laboratory tests (e.g., serology) that may become validated by laboratory confirmation.

Florida

On October 2, the Palm Beach County Health Department (PBCHD) and the Florida Department of Health (FDOH) were notified of a possible anthrax case in Palm Beach County. The suspected case was identified when a gram stain of cerebrospinal fluid (CSF) revealed a gram-positive bacilli. An epidemiologic investigation was initiated by FDOH, PBCHD, and the FDOH state laboratory. The state laboratory and CDC confirmed *B. anthracis* from a culture of CSF on October 4. Later the same day, FDOH and CDC epidemiologists and laboratory workers arrived in Palm Beach County to assist PBCHD with the investigation. As of October 16, two confirmed cases of inhalational anthrax have been identified.

The index patient was a 63-year-old male resident of Palm Beach County who sought medical care at a local hospital on October 2 with fever and altered mental status. Despite antibiotic therapy, his clinical condition deteriorated rapidly, and he died on October 5. An autopsy performed on October 6 confirmed the cause of death as inhalational anthrax. An investigation revealed no obvious exposures to *B. anthracis*.

On October 1, the second patient, a 73-year-old co-worker of the index patient, was admitted to a local hospital for pneumonia. On October 5, a nasal swab was obtained from the patient that yielded a positive culture for *B. anthracis*.

Subsequent testing revealed positive PCR tests for *B. anthracis* in hemorrhagic pleural fluid and reactive serologic tests. The patient remains hospitalized on antibiotic therapy. Enhanced case finding and retrospective and prospective surveillance systems were initiated in Palm Beach, and surrounding counties. Environmental assessments and sampling were performed at the index patient's home, work site, and travel destinations for the 60 days preceding symptom onset. Environmental sampling revealed *B. anthracis* contamination of the work site, specifically implicating mail or package delivery. Environmental samples of other locations the patient visited, including extensive sampling of his home, were negative.

Questionnaires were administered to employees at the index patient's work site. Postexposure prophylaxis was administered, and nasal swabs were obtained from those with exposure to the work site for >1 hour since August 1. Of 1,075 nasal swabs performed, one was positive for *B. anthracis*. Environmental and co-worker testing indicated contamination of specific locations at the work site. The investigation and environmental sampling are ongoing.

New York

On October 9, the New York City Department of Health notified CDC of a person with a skin lesion consistent with cutaneous anthrax. CDC sent a team to New York City to provide epidemiologic and laboratory support to local health officials. As of October 16, two persons with confirmed cases of cutaneous anthrax have been identified. One person with confirmed anthrax was a 38-year-old woman who had handled a suspicious letter postmarked September 18 at her workplace. The letter contained a powder that subsequently was confirmed to contain *B. anthracis*. On September 25, the patient had a raised lesion on the chest, which over the next 3 days developed surrounding erythema and edema. By September 29, the patient developed malaise and headache. On October 1, a clinician examined the patient and described an approximately 5 cm long oval-shaped lesion with a raised border, small satellite vesicles, and profound edema. The lesion was nonpainful and was associated with left cervical lymphadenopathy. Serous fluid from the lesion was obtained and was negative by gram stain and culture. The patient was prescribed oral ciprofloxacin. Over the next several days, the lesion developed a black eschar, and a biopsy was obtained and sent to CDC for testing. The tissue was positive by immunohistochemical staining for the cell wall antigen of *B. anthracis*.

The other person with confirmed cutaneous anthrax was a 7-month-old infant who visited his mother's workplace on September 28. The next day, the infant had an apparently nontender, massively edematous, weeping skin lesion on his left arm; he was treated with intravenous antibiotics. Over the next several days, the lesion became ulcerative and developed a black eschar; clinicians presumptively attributed the lesion to a spider bite. The infant's clinical course was complicated by hemolytic anemia and thrombocytopenia, requiring intensive care. The diagnosis of cutaneous anthrax was first considered on October 12 after the announcement of the other confirmed anthrax case in New York City. A serum specimen collected on October 2 was positive for *B. anthracis* by PCR testing at CDC; a skin biopsy obtained on October 13 was positive by immunohistochemical staining at CDC for the cell wall antigen of *B. anthracis.* No suspicious letter with powder was identified at the mother's workplace. Both patients were treated with ciprofloxacin and are clinically improving.

B. anthracis grew from swabs (two nasal and one facial skin swab) from three other persons, suggesting exposure to anthrax. One of the exposures was in a law enforcement officer who brought the letter containing *B. anthracis* from the index patient's workplace to the receiving laboratory. The other two exposures were in technicians who had processed the letter in the laboratory. Environmental sampling in both workplaces is ongoing and investigations of other exposed persons continue.

Reported by: L Bush, MD, Atlantis; J Malecki, MD, Palm Beach County Health Dept, Palm Beach; S Wiersma, MD, State Epidemiologist, Florida Dept of Health. K Cahill, MD, R Fried, MD; M Grossman, MD, Columbia Presbyterian Medical Center; W Borkowsky, MD, New York Univ Medical Center, New York, New York; New York City Dept of Health. National Center for Infectious Diseases; and EIS officers, CDC.

Editorial Note:

The findings in this report indicate that four confirmed cases of anthrax have resulted from intentional delivery of *B. anthracis* spores through mailed letters or packages. These are the first confirmed cases of anthrax associated with intentional exposure in the United States and represent a new public health threat.

Anthrax is an acute infectious disease caused by the spore-forming bacterium *B. anthracis*. It occurs most frequently as an epizootic or enzootic disease of herbivores (e.g., cattle, goats, or sheep) that acquire spores from direct contact with contaminated soil. Humans usually become infected through direct contact with *B. anthracis* spores from infected animals or their products (e.g., goat hair), resulting in cutaneous anthrax (2) (Box 1). Inhalational and gastrointestinal are other forms of the disease in the natural setting (*4,5*). Human-to-human transmission has not been documented.

Clinical laboratorians should be alert to the presence of *Bacillus* species in patient specimens. In particular, laboratorians should suspect *B. anthracis* when the specimen is from a previously healthy patient with a rapidly progressive respiratory illness or a cutaneous ulcer. If *B. anthracis* is suspected, laboratories should immediately notify the health-care provider and local and state public health staff. For rapid identification of *B. anthracis*, state and local health departments should access the Laboratory Response Network for Bioterrorism (LRN). LRN links state and local public health laboratories with advanced capacity laboratories---including clinical, military, veterinary, agricultural, water, and food-testing laboratories. Laboratorians should contact their state public health laboratory to identify their local LRN representative.

Postexposure prophylaxis is indicated to prevent inhalational anthrax after a confirmed or suspected aerosol exposure. When no information is available about the antimicrobial susceptibility of the implicated strain of *B. anthracis*, initial therapy with ciprofloxacin or doxycycline is recommended for adults and children (Table 1). Use of tetracyclines and fluoroquinolones in children has adverse effects. The risks for these adverse effects must be weighed carefully against the risk for developing life-threatening disease. As soon as penicillin susceptibility of the organism has been confirmed, prophylactic therapy for children should be changed to oral amoxicillin 80 mg/kg of body mass per day divided every 8 hours (not to exceed 500 mg three times daily). *B. anthracis* is not susceptible to cephalosporins or to trimethoprim/sulfamethoxazole, and these agents should not be used for prophylaxis.

CDC is assisting other states and local areas in assessing anthrax exposures. Additional information about anthrax and the public health response is available at <http://www.bt.cdc.gov>. This information was current as of 4 p.m., eastern daylight time, October 17, 2001.

References

1. CDC. Ongoing investigation of anthrax---Florida, October 2001. MMWR 2001;50:877.
2. CDC. Human anthrax associated with an epizootic among livestock---North Dakota, 2000. MMWR 2001;50:677--80.
3. Ashford DA, Rotz LD, Perkins BA. Use of anthrax vaccine in the United States: recommendations of the Advisory Committee on Immunization Practice (ACIP). MMWR 2000;49(no. RR-15).
4. Brachman PS. Inhalational anthrax. Ann NY Acad Sci 1980;353:83--93.
5. Brachman PS, Kaufmann A. Anthrax. In: Evans AS, Brachman PS, eds. Bacterial infections of humans. New York, New York: Plenum Medical Book Company, 1998.

- *Cutaneous* illness is characterized by a skin lesion evolving from a papule, through a vesicular stage, to a depressed black eschar; edema, erythema, or necrosis without ulceration may be present. *Inhalational* illness is characterized by a brief prodrome resembling a "nonspecific febrile" illness that rapidly progresses to a fulminant illness with signs of sepsis and/or respiratory failure, often with radiographic evidence of mediastinal widening; signs of bacterial meningitis may be present. *Gastrointestinal* illness is characterized by severe abdominal pain usually accompanied by bloody vomiting or diarrhea followed by fever and signs of septicemia.

BOX 1. Clinical forms of anthrax
Clinical Forms of Anthrax
The following clinical descriptions of anthrax are based on experience in adults. The clinical presentation of anthrax in infants is not well defined.
Inhalational. Inhalational anthrax begins with a brief prodrome resembling a viral respiratory illness followed by development of hypoxia and dyspnea, with radiographic evidence of mediastinal widening. Inhalational anthrax is the most lethal form of anthrax and results from inspiration of 8,000--50,000 spores of *Bacillus anthracis* (*3*). The incubation period of inhalational anthrax among humans typically ranges from 1--7 days but may be possibly up to 60 days. Host factors, dose of exposure, and chemoprophylaxis may affect the duration of the incubation period. Initial symptoms include mild fever, muscle aches, and malaise and may progress to respiratory failure and shock; meningitis frequently develops. Case-fatality estimates for inhalational anthrax are extremely high, even with all possible supportive care including appropriate antibiotics.
Cutaneous. Cutaneous anthrax is characterized by a skin lesion evolving from a papule, through a vesicular stage, to a depressed black eschar. The incubation period ranges from 1--12 days. The lesion is usually painless, but patients also may have fever, malaise, headache, and regional lymphadenopathy. The case fatality rate for cutaneous anthrax is 20% without, and <1% with, antibiotic treatment.

Gastrointestinal. Gastrointestinal anthrax is characterized by severe abdominal pain followed by fever and signs of septicemia. This form of anthrax usually follows after eating raw or undercooked contaminated meat and can have an incubation period of 1--7 days. An oropharyngeal and an abdominal form of the disease have been described. Involvement of the pharynx is usually characterized by lesions at the base of the tongue, dysphagia, fever, and regional lymphadenopathy. Lower bowel inflammation typically causes nausea, loss of appetite, and fever followed by abdominal pain, hematemesis, and bloody diarrhea. The case-fatality rate is estimated to be 25%--60%. The effect of early antibiotic treatment on the case-fatality rate is not established.

Table 1

Use of trade names and commercial sources is for identification only and does not imply endorsement by the U.S. Department of Health and Human Services.

References to non-CDC sites on the Internet are provided as a service to *MMWR* readers and do not constitute or imply endorsement of these organizations or their programs by CDC or the U.S. Department of Health and Human Services. CDC is not responsible for the content of pages found at these sites.

Appendix 3

Excerpts from Memoranda by Biological Warfare Epidemiologist Meryl Nass, M.D., September-October 2001

Anthrax Vaccine Home Page – www.anthraxvaccine.org
Meryl Nass, M.D., 124 Wardtown Road, Freeport, Maine 04032
Telephone: 207-865-7000.

<u>**September 20, 2001 Update**</u>
The Vaccine

If anthrax is used for bioterrorism, the existing vaccine may or may not be effective. In the one human study ever done of any anthrax vaccine, the vaccine was about 70% effective at preventing anthrax infections. The current vaccine's effectiveness has not been tested in humans. Although it was 95% effective in monkeys, there are reasons to believe monkeys respond to it better than humans. Antibiotics (doxycycline and ciprofloxacin) prevented anthrax in 80% and 90% of a small number of monkeys. But both antibiotics and vaccines can be defeated using widely known genetic engineering techniques to create resistant anthrax strains, or specially selecting naturally occurring anthrax strains.

Anthrax experts in the past have felt that antibiotics are an excellent prophylactic measure, but that vaccines will add to their protection when given *following* an exposure, based on animal experiments.

The vaccine presently available has caused longlasting medical illness in a significant proportion of those who receive it. All existing doses are currently under quarantine by FDA for manufacturing lapses. Even if FDA decides the bioterrorism risk is real and releases the quarantined vaccine for military or civilian use, the manufacturing lapses and risk of chronic illness *remain*.

If the antibiotics are effective (this depends on the strain of anthrax employed), one has time to consider use of the vaccine afterward. If antibiotics are not effective, then the vaccine may be lifesaving, or may be ineffective. But I suspect that 10-35% of vaccine recipients develop illnesses resembling chronic fatigue syndrome, fibromyalgia, multiple chemical sensitivity, autoimmune illnesses, and/or neuropathies: also known as "Gulf War Syndrome." This is the tradeoff you are making when receiving this vaccine.

Exposure

Anthrax does NOT spread from person to person. It ONLY affects those who breathe in the spores when first released. There is only a tiny risk from spores that are re-aerosolized later. Therefore, if you are not in the immediate area of release, or in a narrow path where spores of sufficient quantity are carried by the wind (it requires tens of thousands to millions of spores to cause infection) you will not be affected.

Antibiotics

One can, however, take antibiotics *in advance of* an attack, and still get their benefit if an anthrax attack were to occur. Personally, I have antibiotics handy, but will use them only if attack appears imminent or has occurred. If vaccine is made available, you will never find me lining up for my dose...by the way, there are six initial doses and then one-two yearly booster shots. Protection, you see, does not come quickly, nor easily.

Although dose recommendations for antibiotic therapy exist, they are theoretical, and do not reflect actual experience in humans. Cephalosporins are the only antibiotic class to which anthrax is naturally resistant. So use a high normal dose for a long duration (1-6 months because ungerminated spores can persist in the lungs longterm and germinate following antibiotic cessation): post exposure, when the organism can be cultured, the recommendations can be refined.

One other theoretical consideration is that doxycycline and cipro have been the recommended drugs for anthrax for a decade, and therefore specific resistance to those two may have been added to enhance virulence. This might lead you to choose a second or even third antibiotic to which the organism is less likely to be resistant.

The Initial Response to Anthrax Attacks

October 14, 2001 Update: Response to two reported anthrax attacks suboptimal. What can be improved?

Coming up with more effective responses to the anthrax threat requires a solid understanding of the unique characteristics of anthrax, how it is like and unlike other pathogens for which we have very effective answers.

This is important both to save lives, but also to avoid panic. People are afraid when they do not know what to expect, and do not know how to properly protect themselves. The public and the doctors caring for them have to be

92

educated on anthrax asap. These are my suggestions for expediting the evaluation of anthrax "events" and the prophylactic treatment of those exposed.

I do not wish to be alarmist, but now that the anthrax genie is out of the bottle, we could be seeing a very large number of anthrax scares ahead. I have composed the following very quickly in hopes that it will help us to be optimally prepared.

1. It takes the inhalation of hundreds of thousands to millions of spores of anthrax to cause the disease inhalation anthrax, with the possible exception of people with immune deficiencies, for whom less spores might lead to illness. Fewer spores do not cause illness; the immune system seems to readily defend against them. This is presumably why 5 others in Florida have now been found with anti-anthrax antibodies, but were not ill. In goat hair mills, where workers were daily exposed to anthrax spores, some developed antibodies and some did not. (Our antibody (ELISA) tests may not detect all antibodies to anthrax.)

2. If there were enough spores inhaled in Florida to kill one worker, then there must have been millions more in the office. Other workers would have therefore had spores on clothes, shoes, hair. At this time, I would suggest these items be washed (see comments on washing below) or brushed out, outdoors. There would have been spores on the desks, floors, and in the indoor air. Proper sampling of the environment should have detected these spores, and should have provided an estimate of the magnitude of the exposure. This would have permitted an extrapolation of the risk to individuals working in the office, elsewhere in the building, and in the neighborhood of the building. It would have allowed appropriate antibiotic prescribing for those at risk, who could have been observed carefully and received additional investigations that would be appropriate to their risk.

3. Instead, workers with only gloves on did some environmental sampling when the first case was diagnosed, and employees were allowed to remain in the building for an additional week, where they would have received further exposure to anthrax spores. The environmental samples and nasal swabs were all said to be negative, apart from one person and one computer keyboard. This is simply not possible. Almost fifty years ago, an electrician at Fort Detrick died after doing some work in a building where anthrax research was conducted. Samples taken then (1950s) showed that the building was grossly contaminated, with anthrax spores all over. Why was the Florida sampling so much less sensitive than the sampling that took place in the 1950s? Why did it take authorities a week to figure out that the other employees were also exposed, and that the building was contaminated?

4. At NBC New York, the FBI was notified of a suspicious letter on September 25, but did not test it "until at least two weeks later, when a private doctor city public health officials..." (Steinhauer J and Dwyer J. FBI Did Not Test Letter to NBC or Immediately Notify City Hall. NY Times October 13, 2001. Page A1.) I'm guessing that the spate of hoaxes has rapidly overwhelmed the FBI's ability to deal with each, and overwhelmed their forensic lab's capability. Hoaxes may also be a strategy of a terrorist. Remember how the anti-ballistic missile program has been criticized for its inability to deal with thousands of dummy missiles which could provide cover for a small number of "real" missiles? We may be seeing the same thing now. There is one simple answer: the techniques for doing forensic investigation of suspect materials need to be shared with state and local laboratories, so that these efforts can be decentralized. Then sufficient personnel can be made available to do adequate testing. It may be that of the billions now allotted for terrorism, money should be spent training lab technicians in these techniques, and in training more lab technicians, since we do not know for how long US citizens will be at risk of bioterrorism exposures.

5. How do you test for anthrax, when a variety of tests are available with varying specificities and sensitivities? Well, first of all, you do not allow human beings to be the canaries in the mineshaft, which happened in NYC. Tests of environmental samples can be performed in hours, not days, which is how long cultures take to identify an organism. Cultures are needed for antibiotic sensitivity testing, but the <u>diagnosis of exposure</u> in cases of anthrax needs to be made more quickly, in order to avoid loss of lives.

6. The first test to be done should be extremely sensitive; it does not need to have extreme specificity. The follow-on tests can be more specific. PCR testing fits this bill. If PCR is positive, then aggressive environmental samples, nasal swabs, sputum, blood, cerebrospinal fluid in suspected meningitis cases can be obtained. If a massive exposure has occurred, case-finding is done to identify all those potentially exposed. All are treated with antibiotics prior to any signs of illness. I would propose consideration of bronchoalveolar lavage in highly exposed patients. This procedure has never been reported in anthrax exposures, because there have been no reported exposures since the technique came into clinical practice. However, it might be capable of removing large numbers of spores, and it might also provide an estimate of the risk for the patient and others who had similar levels of exposure, based on the amount of spores recovered from the lungs. We should learn whether this procedure is likely to be helpful.

7. Additional tests could be done as well. One described in the October 13 NY Times page B8 quoted Tom O'Brien of Tetracore, in Gaithersburg, MD is an antigen test which is supplied to federal and local authorities, and can

be performed in 15 minutes. Four groups described different prototype anthrax identification systems for air and other environmental samples at the 1998 international anthrax meeting in the UK. Someone needs to review all these devices and determine their sensitivity and specificity for environmental samples, and make the most promising devices available to local authorities for widespread air/environmental sampling asap. It may be that the US will have to live with biosensors in public places, now that the anthrax genie is out of the bottle. Not a pleasing option, but one that might provide the lead time needed to treat people during that important window: after exposure, but before serious illness has developed.

8. <u>Treatment</u>: not so simple as popping a cipro tablet twice a day. First off, the risks involved in taking an antibiotic that you don't need for a few days or weeks are really not that large. However, if everyone starts taking antibiotics in advance of any known exposures, there will not be enough available in 6 or 12 months, and then the terrorists can play havoc with us. If it makes you feel more secure, keep a week or two of any antibiotic on hand. The Florida anthrax strain was reported to be sensitive to just about every oral antibiotic, including penicillins, tetracyclines and quinolones such as ciprofloxiacin. The problem is this: we do not know how long you will need to take them, and we do not know if all the anthrax held by terrorists will be antibiotic sensitive, as the Florida strain apparently was. Monkey experiments showed that the animals survived lethal anthrax exposures when antibiotics were provided within 24 hours following exposure, but that some died when antibiotics were stopped, after a month or more. So how long do you take them for? Personally, I would take them for at least six months, if that were the only treatment I had. I would only know which to take after antibiotic sensitivity testing had been done. I might start with doxycycline, since I am pen allergic and it is inexpensive, and saved 9 out of 10 monkeys. Cipro saved 8 out of 10, if memory serves. Given the small number of animals tested, there is no difference in effectiveness between these two. Neither drug is ideal for children or pregnant women, who should receive a macrolide, penicillin or sulfa drug. The environmental sampling, if done properly, should alert you to your own level of exposure, and therefore your risk. If I inhaled 100 spores, I would not take anything. The data are that good on chronic occupational exposures in contaminated environments, that I am assured I would not become ill.

9. Methods for inactivating spores in the environment need to be provided to the public. On Scotland's Gruinard Island, contaminated with anthrax for 45 years after experiments performed with anthrax during World War Two, anthrax was killed after contaminated areas were defoliated, and a dilute solution of formaldehyde in seawater was sprayed on the land. Bleach has also been used, but I do not know the concentration needed or the amount of time required in which the solution must be in contact with the spores.

10. Detergents can <u>increase</u> the virulence of anthrax spores, and thereby decrease the number needed to cause disease. It may be that the addition of detergents at the Manchester NH goat hair mill where the US' only epidemic of inhalation anthrax occurred (5 cases in 1957), was the cause of the epidemic. This increasing of spore virulence by detergent was described in a paper by JM Barnes: "The development of anthrax following the administration of spores by inhalation." British J Experimental Pathology 1947, vol 28, pp385-94. I would therefore <u>not</u> wash contaminated clothes or surfaces with detergents, until we have been informed exactly what to use and what not to use, by those who have done the appropriate experiments at Fort Detrick Maryland or Porton Down in the UK.

11. What about masks? What about envelopes? What about opening packages? Obviously, if you are concerned, open things in such a way as to prevent widespread dissemination of contents, like opening with scissors instead of ripping. Better yet, give it to the authorities. Open things so that you are upwind of them. Don't inhale while opening, if you feel you need to go to these lengths. Besides gas masks, there are other medical masks which are cheap and easy and might be helpful. Again, we need the information from authorities who have tested the masks to learn exactly what types of protection they provide. Do they keep out 98% of particulates of the one to five micron size? If so, that would be a good mask for opening letters that might contain anthrax spores, if you work in the media or a mailroom/post office.

12. New treatment methodologies need to be put into place asap. Antiserum needs to be produced in the US now, as a potentially life-saving treatment for late-diagnosed cases. Existing stocks should be sought from China and possibly Russia. (See the October 14, 2001 Chicago Tribune: US Speeds Vaccine Creation, Research by Peter Gorner.) Monoclonal antibodies, which are actively being researched, need to be made available for experimental use, in the event they are needed for life-threatening cases of anthrax. (See the October 12, 2001 Reuters article: University of Texas Team Works on Anthrax Treatment.)

Bottom Line:

1. Environmental sampling needs to be made more accurate, using known techniques, and more widespread. <u>Forensic testing of samples needs to be decentralized</u>, so it can be done in a timely manner, and so the federal authorities are not overwhelmed. The federal government should pay the salaries of additional technicians in every state and possibly in large hospitals, who would be trained as forensic experts, and provide the materials and methodologies used by our federal experts at Fort Detrick, CDC and the FBI, among others.

2. Methods which go from most highly sensitive to most highly specific need to be used, in the proper order, so potential anthrax cases can be identified and treated in a timely manner. This means that existing tests that take hours, not days, need to be the primary ones used.

3. <u>All</u> questionable materials must be tested using sensitive techniques. We do not yet know how to select those which can be ignored.

4. The public needs to be reassured that in fact, the government will address these incidents promptly and effectively, so that the public is not responsible for its own antibiotics and treatment strategies.

5. Biosensors in development need to be assessed now, and the best ones need to be put into mass production.

6. Pharmaceutical companies should increase production of a variety of antibiotics, and government stockpiles of these materials should increase.

7. Novel approaches to treatment should be investigated and prepared or obtained in advance. This might include antiserum, monoclonal antibodies, and other materials currently being developed. The utility of bronchoalveolar lavage in monkeys should be investigated. The sensitivity of nasal swab testing, sputum, urine and blood antigen tests, stains and cultures should be assessed in animal models immediately.

8. Information on safe methods for inactivating spores found in or on contaminated clothes, surfaces and other environmental materials should be provided to the public immediately.

9. Information on cheap masks, like those worn by lab techs working under hoods, that have high efficacy for anthrax, should be provided to the public. Production should be increased.

October 21 Update - Current Anthrax Situation

- More envelopes are being discovered with anthrax spores.
- Government spokespersons equivocate on whether the materials are "weapons grade."
- Better detection of anthrax spores appears to be taking place, but slowly.
- Congressional office buildings have been shut down for decontamination, but the methods for doing so have not been discussed.
- Some other buildings that have received anthrax-containing letters remain open.

- A case of inhalation anthrax has been diagnosed in a Washington DC postal worker

Issues that need to be addressed regarding the bioterrorism response include the following:

1. Are the anthrax-containing envelopes an initial tease, or warning? They are a good way to disseminate small quantities, while avoiding identification of the sender. But what may be ahead? Spores in ventilation systems? Spores at sports events or where there are dense population concentrations? Thousands or millions of letters containing anthrax? How will we know in time, and how will we decontaminate ventilation systems, electronics, sports arenas, soil, etc.?

2. At the present time, public health authorities have continued to use (primarily cutaneous) human anthrax cases as the harbingers of anthrax dissemination. Cutaneous infections require many fewer spores to induce illness, compared to inhalation anthrax. The infected individuals are serving as the "canaries in the mineshaft" who warn that anthrax is present. If the extent of spore dissemination increases (higher concentrations in ambient air from envelopes, or through other means) then the *inhalation cases* will serve as the canaries, and there will be many fatalities.

3. I will continue to harp on the need for *accurate and rapid sampling of the environment* as the most important (by far) technology needed to deal with the offensive use of anthrax. There are likely to be many more envelopes that have already dispersed anthrax spores, but have not been identified yet, because there have (so far) been no cases of illness related to those envelopes, and spores were not seen by the person(s) handling the mail. This means that anthrax spores may be contaminating a number of environments in which they have not been detected. We may not see cases until small animals, children, or people with immune system impairment become exposed in those environments.

4. Only by *identifying an environment contaminated with anthrax before illness appears* are we likely to effectively treat inhalation cases.

5. Only by identifying these environments can we remove people from the environment and protect them from further exposure.

6. *It is possible that we will not be able to do a complete clean up of contaminated environments, for the time being*. There has not been a great deal of research into how to clean up homes and offices, for example. Gruinard Island, off the coast of Scotland, was

decontaminated 45 years after it was used as a test area for anthrax during World War II. During those 45 years, humans and animals were barred from the island. Ten acres were decontaminated: this required defoliating the area, using 200 tons of 37% formaldehyde, diluted in seawater, that was sprayed over the area, and then additional formaldehyde was re-sprayed after deep soil sampling revealed persistent organisms.

7. What else works to kill anthrax spores, which can remain viable for decades or hundreds or years? Bleach, which must be in contact with spores for at least 2 minutes. Paraformaldehyde gas, glutaraldehyde, hydrogen peroxide and peracetic acid also work, and need to be in contact with spores for at least as long. But these materials can be corrosive and are not appropriate for homes and offices, though they can be used to decontaminate most laboratories. Spores can be boiled; the standard recommendation has been to keep the water at a rolling boil at least 10 minutes to kill spores of any pathogen. Steam also kills spores in from 1 to 10 minutes. In goat hair mills, the goat hair was treated at 170 degrees Fahrenheit for 15 minutes, but many spores retained their viability after this treatment. Moist heat works much better than dry heat. Fumigation can be performed with ethylene or propylene oxides, or paraformaldehyde gas.

8. I hope you can tell from this that I do not know a completely safe and effective way to perform decontamination. This needs to be an area of intensive investigation now. **Dr. Alibek has suggested that methods used for decontamination in Sverdlovsk in 1979 (washing trees and houses, and paving dirt roads), may have re-aerosolized anthrax spores, and that this may have _increased_ the number of cases of inhalation anthrax.**

9. Dr. Ken Alibek suggested steam ironing letters before opening, which sounds like a good idea. Put a cloth between the iron and the letter. We need to know more about the temperature setting and how long the iron needs to be in contact with the letter.

10. The bottom line is that spores are odorless, tasteless, and invisible, individually. In a worst case scenario, up to one trillion spores (1,000,000,000,000) might be present in one gram of material. One gram can be contained easily within a one-ounce (28 gram) letter. It theoretically could contain a million lethal doses, if the majority of the spores were viable, of the right size, and dispersed easily without clumping.

11. **What is a lethal dose of spores?** The reason why you may read a variety of different estimates for this number is because a) there are no human-derived data, and b) there are a variety of factors that

impact the answer. There are many animal experiments, and those results are surprising at times. It also depends on the virulence of the anthrax strain used, the amount of air you inhale (during exercise, you breathe in several times as much air as you do at rest), the % of viable spores, the distribution of size of spores, whether the spores easily separate from each other, and your own inherent immune system function. Thus the number might range from 10,000 spores to many millions. Animal tests of a sample from a letter should give us a rough idea of how virulent the potion is, and what a lethal dose might be.

12. Here are some animal data for lethal doses (LD50) of anthrax spores by subcutaneous injection and inhalation (from JM Barnes). This shows why there are so many cutaneous cases, compared to inhalation cases.

Species	# spores injected	# spores inhaled
Rabbit	100-1000	600,000
Guinea Pig	100-1000	370,000
Mouse	10-100	1,400,000

13. Another experiment in pigs: each of 50 pigs was fed from 10 million to 10 billion Ames strain spores (C Redmond et al.) Only 2 of the pigs died (4% of the total) and two others had anthrax isolated from blood, but survived. By 21 days after feeding the spores, the majority of pigs had developed antibodies to anthrax, indicating that they became infected and recovered. Humans, like pigs, are probably relatively resistant to anthrax, compared to many other species.

14. How do we know antiserum is likely to be protective? Mice, which are notoriously hard to protect against anthrax with vaccines, were given antiserum and then exposed to anthrax. The survival of mice given two different antisera was 80% at two weeks post exposure for both groups, while those given control sera had a 0% or 10% survival rate (RJ Beedham et al).

15. It remains very important to keep one's exposure to anthrax spores to a minimum, particularly if you work in a high risk industry, such as the postal service, UPS, Fedex, media or politics. Although I earlier advised against gas masks, I have come to believe ***there is a role for appropriate, well-fitted masks that have demonstrated efficacy in preventing inhalation of particles of the 0.5 to 5.0 micron size.*** My hope is that once environmental sensors are used widely, we will be able to discard masks. For now, if you feel there has been an exposure, or if you are trying to avoid exposure at a high risk occupation, HEPA dust masks (such as 3M Corp has sold for tuberculosis prophylaxis) may be useful. The more HEPA sheets in the mask, the better it will filter. These masks have not been tested for

anthrax or other bioterrorism exposures, so 3M cannot market them for this purpose. However, such masks ought to keep out 95-99% of particles in the desired size range, and could be used for "high risk" activities such as opening mail. Gloves would also decrease one's exposure to spores, but must be discarded after use, or washed after use in order to reuse them.

16. Again, let me emphasize that a variety of soaps and detergents have been tested and were found to *increase* spore virulence by up to a factor of 16. That means the spores could be made 16 times as virulent, because soaps may make them easier to disperse as individual particles. For now, **wash only in water first to remove spores;** you can then use soap when the spores are down the drain.

17. There are many methodologies for identifying spores in the environment. I have collected a large number of articles on this subject, and will discuss what looks promising, and the differences between the methods, in a subsequent update. I continue to believe that PCR testing, because of its sensitivity and rapidity, should be the initial test done, with the understanding that some false positives will result, but no anthrax exposures will be missed, as long as sampling is adequate. I have spoken at length to Tom O'Brien of Tetracore, in Gaithersburg, MD. His company has some very promising PCR and immunoassays for anthrax that can be completed in under 12 hours, and can detect as few as 100 cfu (viable spores) per milliliter of material.

18. Diagnosing exposure in people is not that easy. Although obtaining nasal swabs is a simple procedure to perform, one study shows that the spores rapidly disappear from the nose after exposure, suggesting that swabs are only likely to be positive within 24 hours of contact. Thus sensitivity may be very low, and swabs will give you many false negative results.

19. Treatment is another question. I have suggested that many other antibiotics are as good or better than ciprofloxacin. Doxycycline, for instance, will also work for plague, tularemia and brucella, and effectiveness for all these other potential biowarfare pathogens has not been established for cipro.

20. The duration of antibiotic treatment needed remains uncertain. It is not clear if those currently being treated are being helped by antibiotics, or would not have become ill anyway. Antibody titers will tell if you successfully fought off anthrax. Although CDC Deputy Director David Fleming said that a four-fold rise in antibody titer is needed to confirm recent anthrax infection, this is not necessarily the case. Because anthrax is so rare, one positive antibody titer (by

ELISA) should be adequate to make the diagnosis, as long as the ELISA test is accurate.

21. A pathologist called me today regarding an autopsy of a possible anthrax case. Autopsies can be a problem; in animals, when the animal is opened, spores form and are released. This could contaminate the autopsy suite. There may be temperatures in which this does not occur, but I don't know that for sure. I recommended instead, that blood, CSF and mediastinal fluid be sampled for the presence of the relatively unique-appearing gram positive fat rods of anthrax. This might save you from having to do a whole autopsy.

22. How to protect pets? The animal vaccine works quite well though it may require yearly boosters (there is little data on how frequently they must be given).

23. I guess my take home message is that, unlike other pathogens, which live in the environment for minutes to, at most, days, these spores last nearly forever. Contamination does not resolve with time, although if spores are kicked up inside buildings, they may disperse to less infectious levels. ***Outdoors, the spores tend to stick to the soil components and do not easily re-aerosolize. However, that may not be the case for indoor spore accumulations.*** First responders, affected workers, and others who may be in the vicinity of an anthrax event should behave as if there are invisible, potentially lethal spores everywhere: on surfaces, floors, your computer and desk, your person, walls and ceilings. This requires an entirely new mindset for dealing with infectious emergencies.

Meryl Nass, MD
www.anthraxvaccine.org